THE
BACK
SUFFERERS'
POCKET GUIDE

D1549805

700036912755

THE
BACK
SUFFERERS'
POCKET GUIDE

SARAH KEY
& VICKY ROBERTS

Vermilion
LONDON

1 3 5 7 9 10 8 6 4 2

Published in 2010 by Vermilion, an imprint of Ebury Publishing

Ebury Publishing is a Random House Group company

Text copyright © Sarah Key and Vicky Roberts 2010
Illustrations copyright © Robert Harvey 2010

Sarah Key and Vicky Roberts have asserted their right to be identified as the authors
of this Work in accordance with the Copyright, Designs and Patents Act 1988.

The Random House Group Limited Reg. No. 954009

Addresses for companies within the Random House Group can be found at
www.rbooks.co.uk

A CIP catalogue record for this book is available from the British Library

The Random House Group Limited supports The Forest Stewardship
Council (FSC), the leading international forest certification organisation.
All our titles that are printed on Greenpeace approved FSC certified paper
carry the FSC logo. Our paper procurement policy can be found
at www.rbooks.co.uk/environment

Printed and bound in Great Britain by CPI Cox & Wyman, Reading, RG1 8EX

ISBN 9780091929497

Copies are available at special rates for bulk orders.
Contact the sales development team on 020 7840 8487 for more information.

To buy books by your favourite authors and register for offers, visit
www.rbooks.co.uk

The information in this book has been compiled by way of general guidance in
relation to the specific subjects addressed, but is not a substitute and not to be
relied on for medical, healthcare, pharmaceutical or other professional advice on
specific circumstances and in specific locations. Please consult your GP before
changing, stopping or starting any medical treatment. So far as the authors are
aware, the information given is correct and up to date as at December 2009.
Practice, laws and regulations all change, and the reader should obtain up-to-date
professional advice on any such issues. The authors and publishers disclaim,
as far as the law allows, any liability arising directly or indirectly from the
use, or misuse, of the information contained in this book.

CONTENTS

INTRODUCTION

This little book is designed to be a quick and
easy guide to the treatment of back pain.
Providing a concise, easy-to-follow exercise
programme, and packed with helpful hints,
techniques and advice, it will help you take
control of your back problem and restore
you to your former life. *The Back Sufferers'
Pocket Guide* does not take the place of *Sarah
Key's Back Sufferers' Bible,* which covers all
the vitally important details of spinal
function, anatomy and the mechanisms that
go wrong, but is an aide-memoire to be
carried in your pocket or handbag until the
exercises become second nature to you.

Back pain affects 80 per cent of us at some point in our lives, and is the second most popular reason for visiting the GP's surgery. In the UK one in six working days is lost due to back pain, and there are no obvious signs of these alarming statistics improving.

As practising physiotherapists, we see the misery back pain can cause, but we also see the improvements that can result from a combination of simple treatment, minor lifestyle changes and exercise. We hope this book, which has at its core a programme of tried and tested exercises to help you improve the health of your back, will guide you towards a pain-free future.

ONE

IMPORTANT DETAILS OF SPINAL ANATOMY

The back is an intricate jigsaw puzzle of interdependent structures working together with split-second timing to allow us to move safely and comfortably. The spine itself is a column of 24 individual segments called vertebrae. These sit atop a triangular block of bone at the back of the pelvis called the sacrum.

Each vertebra consists of a front and back compartment. When the vertebral segments are stacked vertically, a hole in the middle between the two compartments makes a long, internal tube, which houses the spinal cord hanging down from the base of the brain. Paired spinal nerves branch off the cord and exit the spine on both sides at each spinal level.

The intervertebral discs are slotted between the vertebrae. These are high-pressure, water-filled cushions, which are ingeniously designed as the main shock-absorbing components of the spine. The discs also hold the spinal segments together, and their ability to spring-load the segments as the spine bends brings both flexibility and stability to the column.

At the back of each vertebra, situated on either side and behind each lumbar disc, are two pairs of bony plates called the facet joints. The facet joints are 'movement controllers' rather than weight bearers, and they play a vital role in keeping the spinal segments secure as the low back bends and lowers the upper body.

An intricate arrangement of ligaments helps lash the vertebrae together, while the muscles give us the movement and the dynamic support without which we would crumple over and fall to the floor.

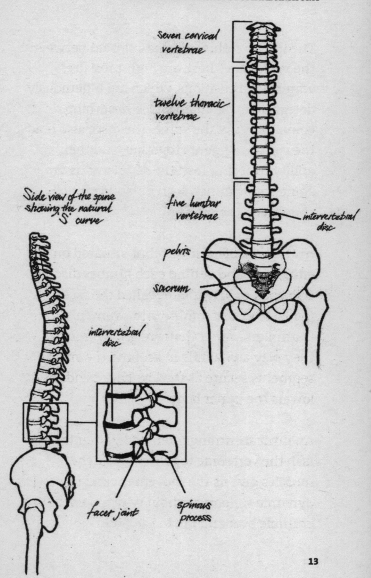

Seven cervical vertebrae

twelve thoracic vertebrae

Side view of the spine showing the natural 'S' curve

five lumbar vertebrae

intervertebral disc

pelvis

sacrum

intervertebral disc

facet joint

spinous process

TWO

THE FIVE STAGES OF BREAKDOWN OF A SPINAL SEGMENT

A spinal segment consists of two vertebrae separated by an intervertebral disc. It is often referred to as a motion segment.

Most spinal conditions develop as part of a sequence of breakdown of a motion segment from simple, easily reversible disorders to more complex and intractable ones. The progressive sequence of degeneration passes through various stages of breakdown, manifesting as five distinct spinal disorders. These are:

Stage 1: A stiff spinal segment

Imagine a stiff spinal segment as a stiff link in a bicycle chain. It occurs when an intervertebral disc loses water and stiffens, and can be caused by several factors, including trauma, sustained compression (long periods of sitting), abnormal postures and abdominal muscle weakness. The back wall of the drier stiff disc becomes susceptible to trauma, often resulting from bending and twisting activities, making it sensitive and loath to stretch. All of this leads to gradual loss of movement between the vertebrae which prevents the disc from

A drier disc cannot hold and circulate as much fluid. As the disc gradually loses height, it makes the spinal segment painful and stiff to movement.

sucking in the fluid needed to keep it pumped up and healthy. The disc then gradually starves, becoming ever drier, stiffer and thinner.

A stiff spinal segment is by far the most common spinal condition and the most likely cause of 'simple back pain'. A stiff segment can sit there for long periods without causing obvious problems, but long term, if the stiffening and disc-thinning is allowed to progress, it can lead to breakdown of the segment through Stages 2 to 5. You will see, in the exercise section of this book, that a large part of self-treatment is aimed at getting sluggish spinal segments moving to thwart this cascade of events playing out.

Stiff spinal segments commonly escape detection through conventional X-ray, CT and MRI scanning, and are best unearthed by palpating with human hands. Symptoms vary from screaming pain and tenderness during the acute (early) phase, through to aching stiffness with gnawing pain, interspersed with high-pitched twinges in the sub-acute phase. In the chronic (later, more long-lasting) phase it usually presents as a deep ache, associated with armour-plated stiffness across the low back.

Stage 2: Facet joint arthropathy

This is the most common development from Stage 1 and occurs where thinning and drying of the disc decreases the clearance between two vertebrae, causing overriding of the bony plates (the facet joints) at the back of the spine. In the early stages, this simply inflames the soft tissues surrounding the joint, but as the facet surfaces gradually bear more weight, there is erosion of the cartilage buffer covering the bone, leading to progressive arthritic changes. An over-arched low back, weak tummy muscles and leg length inequality

As the disc loses height, the facet joints override at the back of the spine, the facet capsule can inflame and irritate the spinal nerve and bring on sciatica.

can also predispose to wear and tear of the facets joints.

The onset of acute inflammation of a facet joint usually follows a wrenching of the spine, and the pain builds slowly. Symptoms of knife-like pain to the side of the low back can be accompanied by flooding pain down the leg (sciatica), caused by irritation of the spinal nerve root caught up in the local inflammation and swelling. Facet joint sciatica is easily set off by changes in position, but recovery from this stage is usually quite rapid. The chronic phase can present as a niggling patch of pain beside the spine, which often craves pummelling from your own fist or fingers to provide relief.

Stage 3: The acute locked back

This is a crisis that results from a momentary lapse in the coordinated control of one of the facet joints. What makes it particularly unnerving is that the hiccup in fine movement occurs at the beginning of an action, usually without warning. Once again, the underlying cause is often the drying and thinning of an intervertebral disc, which reduces its internal pressure and hence its cushioning buoyancy – a bit like a deflated car tyre. The resulting jolt of pain can be of such frightening intensity that it often causes collapse to the floor and a rigid paralysis. The unexpectedness and sheer terror of the episode can leave you with a constant fear of it happening again, and often it seems the back is never the same again.

The uncontrollable, electric jolts of the acute stage may require an injection of a strong painkiller to bring about calm and make the first movements possible. Generally, it is not advisable to go to an A&E Department (where staff are usually at a loss to know what to do) but *it is necessary* to go to bed for at least three days. Bed rest must be coupled with painkillers, anti-inflammatory drugs and muscle relaxants, administered by your doctor, until the armour-plated rigidity of the muscles (muscle spasm) of the low back eases.

Gentle knee-rocking exercises (see page 80) in bed facilitate early recovery and prevent the condition coming and going indefinitely and even progressing to Stage 5.

The reduced disc height and lower disc pressure makes the facets joints harder to control.

Stage 4: The prolapsed 'slipped' disc

This occurs when disc degeneration has progressed to the point where the ball of fluid at the centre (the nucleus) dries out, and load is transferred to the walls of the disc. Excessive twisting or lifting activities can make this unhealthy nuclear material squeeze out through small chinks or fissures in the disc wall, creating pressure and stretch on the pain-sensitive outer layers of the back wall. This can bring on a deep cramping back ache.

If the bulge occurs at one of the back corners of the disc, it may cause pressure on the delicate nerve root nearby and bring on sciatica (leg pain). Occasionally the nucleus ruptures right through the outer wall – imagine the jam in the centre of a doughnut squirting out through the sponge – causing a dramatic increase in leg pain, which lasts until the toxic nuclear material can be absorbed by the bloodstream.

The nerve irritation and inflammation can make any form of leg stretch absolute agony – even the simple act of walking. Sitting brings no relief as it increases spinal compression and causes even more pressure on the nerve. Often side lying, with a pillow between the knees, is the only position of comfort.

> *A degenerated disc nucleus can track out of the centre and create a pressure build-up behind the sensitive outer layers of the disc wall.*

It is worth noting that many of us have discs that are bulging (they would show up on MRI) but causing no trouble at all. Much depends on the location and size of the bulge, and how inflamed everything is around it. Thankfully, disc prolapse is fairly rare. For decades, though, painful backs have been glibly labelled 'slipped disc' for want of a proper understanding of what actually is wrong.

Stage 5: The unstable spinal segment

This is the end condition of a spinal segment breaking down. Here, degeneration has reached the point where the disc and facet joints – which, together, act as the main stabilising structures, supporting and controlling movement of the segment – are unable to hold the segment secure. The vertebra is left loose, like a weak link in the spinal chain, and this makes it susceptible to slipping forward as the spine bends. Although the acute phase is often triggered by strong physical exertion, such as heavy pushing or lifting, or long periods of sustained bending activity, such as gardening, trouble has usually accrued steadily over years of pain and disability. Background factors, such as weight gain and poor fitness levels, often precipitate a crisis period.

A spinal segment becomes unstable as progressive degeneration weakens both the disc and facet joints.

The main sign of instability is a tell-tale wriggle or painful 'catch' as you go to bend, and you are constantly wary of your back painfully giving way. As the generalised muscle stiffness takes over, it can spread through the upper back and neck, even causing headaches. In the chronic phase, when seemingly everyday activities can set off widespread pain and spasm, you lurch between bad and not so bad periods. Your back may start to settle of its own accord, but as the muscle spasm eases and the weak link is exposed, one ill-considered move can catapult you back into an acute phase again, where intolerable leg pain may require surgical intervention.

Segmental instability is the hardest spinal condition to fix yourself, so it's perhaps a good thing it is so rare.

Muscle spasm

Muscle spasm is a reflex triggered by tissue inflammation and pain, and at all the different stages of breakdown it is both friend and foe. Muscle spasm's role is initially protective, where the muscles around an irritable segment clench automatically to minimise movement and let things calm down. In a situation where a back is newly injured, the strong muscle-hold acts like a splint (a bit like a plaster-of-Paris cast on a broken ankle), keeping the damaged area still and perhaps preventing further injury.

Unfortunately, spasm is greatly influenced by fear and anxiety, which can make the mechanism ultra-sensitive and difficult to switch off. Uninterrupted spasm can lock a spinal segment out of the spine's general movement and lead to a vicious cycle, as the spasm clamps pain-sensitive structures and stops the discs evacuating their waste products. This causes more irritation and soreness and may escalate disc breakdown in a matter of weeks. For this reason muscle spasm needs to be addressed as a first priority of treatment, both through medication (see page 44) and 'spinal appeasing' exercises (see exercises 2–5 in Chapter Four).

For a detailed explanation of the process of breakdown, read *Sarah Key's Back Sufferers' Bible*.

THREE

SELF-TREATMENT FOR A BACK PROBLEM

Self-treatment is the key to reversing the physical and physiological changes which are behind most back problems, and requires patience, perseverance and instinct. In most cases disc degeneration is slow, so it follows that all 'therapy' aimed at improving the health of your discs is also likely to be slow. For this reason, self-treatment should be an ongoing process that may need to continue indefinitely. That said, it is important that self-treatment is not viewed as a 'life sentence' of rigorous, time-consuming exercise on a daily basis. Your self-management should be seen as a profoundly satisfying exercise programme which brings newfound freedom to your life. It involves a series of small changes, and does not necessarily mean the avoidance of all strenuous activity.

Reversing the changes behind your problem is ultimately *your* responsibility, but in the early stages of treatment a trained therapist is invaluable at identifying and un-jamming the relevant vertebral segments so they can move more freely. Practitioners of the Sarah Key Method will use their thumbs, the heel of the hand or even the heel of their foot to free up a stiff vertebra as quickly and effortlessly as possible. You then must make the most of this newly acquired freedom through your exercise programme (see Chapter Four), which aims to provide the segmental movement required to stimulate disc metabolism, enhance their fluid exchange, stretch tightened soft tissues and strengthen weak muscles.

To find an accredited practitioner of The Sarah Key Method (APSKM), go to: www.sarahkey.com

To rest or not to rest ...

Bed rest for a limited period can be invaluable in cases where a back is newly injured or there is severe pain due to spasm and inflammation. In such cases, bed rest should be viewed as an important part of the treatment. It:

- eliminates the compression of gravity
- eases muscle spasm, which in turn reduces the clamp on the spinal segments
- improves circulation, which speeds the removal of toxic inflammatory products from both facet joints and discs and encourages healing

How to do 'bed rest' properly

You should rest in bed and aim to stay horizontal, with one pillow (two at most) under your head, and several pillows under your lower legs so that hips and knees are virtually at right angles. Aim to stay relaxed; stave off boredom by reading, listening to music etc., and don't be afraid to change position to side lying – pop a pillow between your knees – and back again. It's fine to get up to visit the bathroom, of course, but go back to bed as soon as possible.

You should always intersperse resting in bed with the gentle 'knees rocking' exercise (exercise 2, page 80) every two hours, or more frequently if you feel inclined. This exercise provides a gentle pumping action, which speeds up the circulation through your lower back and lets the healing begin.

Pillows under your knees help your lower back 'let go', but you can move in bed while lying down as much as you like.

While your back is in crisis, get up by rolling to the edge of the bed and swing your legs over the side while pushing into the bed with both arms to lever yourself up. Remember to keep your tummy braced throughout. To get back into bed again, simply reverse the procedure. Remember, though, that as soon as the crisis has passed, you must return to getting in and out of bed in the normal way. Bending your spine naturally is an essential part of recovery, and getting up from lying down, by effortlessly drawing your upper body forward, is a good example of this. You only roll like a log during an acute phase, while the muscle control is discordant, and the sooner you can progress to moving normally, the more rapidly you will progress. Remember that you risk becoming stuck in invalid mode if you keep protecting the back too much. And finally, remember normal movement is the best therapy of all. It promotes coordinated activity between

muscles and joints, which improves their
circulation, and it makes the spine more
balanced and strong.

Another good way to rest a sore back

Finding a way to switch off muscle spasm and relax a sore back is treatment in its own right, and most backs love it. Here is the way to do it:

Lie on the floor – you can use a yoga mat or a folded towel, if you like – with your hips and knees bent at right angles. Rest your calf muscles on a chair or foot stool.

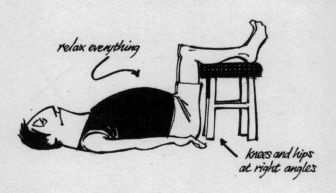

relax everything

knees and hips
at right angles

In this position, your lower back is fully supported, and your muscles can let go. It is fine to pop a small cushion under your head, but don't prop yourself up too high. Now, let the floor take your weight as your legs roll out a little, and just RELAX!

Stay in this position for 10–20 minutes. Bliss!

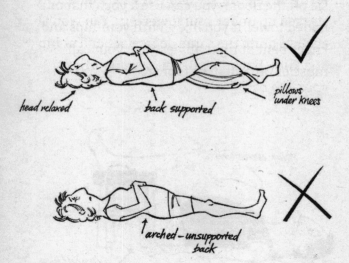

head relaxed   back supported   pillows under knees

arched – unsupported back

Have the stool high enough to take all the weight off your lower back, and let your knees roll out slightly as your legs relax.

If you can't find a suitable chair or stool to rest your legs on, try using several pillows stacked up under your lower legs. You won't achieve quite the same degree of bend at hip and knee, but you will still be supporting your low back.

Medication

There are times when the right medication can work wonders for an acutely painful back. Medication should then be viewed as part of the treatment – a way of releasing you from pain so that you can move on with self-management of your condition.

There are three different categories of medication in common use for back pain:

- painkillers
- muscle relaxants
- anti-inflammatory drugs (NSAIDS)

Your pharmacist can advise you on appropriate over-the-counter medication, but only a qualified medical practitioner can give you prescriptive medicine, which is often stronger and more effective.

Heat

Gentle heat is remarkably good at easing back stiffness, and it also increases blood flow which helps the healing process. If your pain is mild and well managed, try lying on one for 20 minutes at the end of a busy day, or after activity that you know will stiffen you up. If you are undergoing an acute period where your back is irritable and sore, pace yourself through the day and choose to lie down on your heat pad before the pain has geared up. Again, always rock your knees for several minutes after you have been immobile (see exercise 2, page 80), and you will find it easier to get up.

You can buy adhesive, disposable heat pads, which can be marvellous on long journeys. They are discreet enough to be worn under even tightly fitted clothing, and the warmth lasts for up to 8 hours. Follow the instructions on the box to avoid overheating or blistering your skin, and avoid heat rubs when using a heat pad, as combining the two may make your skin overly sensitive.

Ice is usually of little help with back pain.

Sitting

Our modern way of sitting is not ideal for spines. In earlier civilisations people squatted, which is the natural way of pulling out or decompressing the segments at the spine's base. Perching on a conventional seat has the opposite effect. It loads weight through the spine, compresses the lumbar segments and squeezes fluid from the discs. That said, sitting for short periods is not necessarily a bad thing. Compressing the segments helps to evacuate waste products from the discs and actually enhances the turnover of discal fluids. The benefit is lost, however, if you sit for long periods of time (even an hour of uninterrupted sitting is too long),

Sitting in a slumped position compresses the lumbar discs more.

and many of us do! Lengthy periods of sitting depress the metabolic vigour of disc cells which reduces their ability to carry out running repairs. Sustained compression also squeezes too much fluid from the discs, which makes them more leaden.

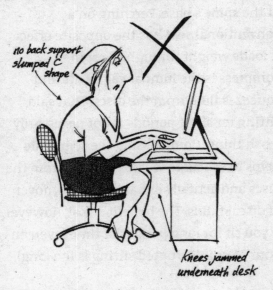

no back support slumped 'C' shape

knees jammed underneath desk

Slumping in a characteristic 'C' shape with tummy muscles off duty increases disc compression even more – so that it takes some time for the full complement of fluid to return. Over the years, as the front of the spinal segments gradually pinch together, the spine becomes permanently tethered forward. Periods of protracted sitting also cause progressive shortening of the ligaments and muscles at the front of the groin, making it difficult to stand fully upright and walk with a full length of stride.

Be aware that the ill-effects of slumped sitting cannot be remedied simply by sitting bolt upright. This action makes your long back muscles tighten up like piano wires, which dramatically increases the compressive forces through your spine. All the more important with acute backs, since people in pain tend to feel they are doing the right thing by trying to sit up as straight as possible.

How to sit properly

The aim is to keep a natural lumbar hollow and preserve a gentle, elongated 'S' bend throughout the spine, head over hips, with effortless and balanced co-contraction of tummy and back muscles. While the back is in rehabilitation mode, the aim is to maintain the lumbar hollow without over-using muscles. This is something that most back pain sufferers find extremely difficult to achieve.

- If your back is in spasm but you can't avoid sitting, a big comfortable bed pillow (feather and down is best) wrapped around the low back will support and cushion your spine, helping to switch off over-active muscles.
- On a long car journey, you may want to tie the pillow in place using a belt at high waist level. Position the belt where your forearm rests when you bend your elbow behind your back at a right angle.
- Remember, during all car journeys you must also take regular breaks. Get out

and stretch and squat (see 'Squatting', page 55). Holding the bumper bar or door frame and leaning back on your heels will help you stretch the bottom of your back more effectively.

- Don't slouch.
- Wherever possible try to adhere to the '20-minute rule': never sit for longer than 20 minutes without a major shift in position (this really means standing up). Move around as much as possible in your seat, elongating your torso skyward, side-bending left to right, and humping and hollowing your lower back by engaging your tummy muscles. You will feel the benefits immediately.
- Practise standing up and squatting at two-hourly intervals during periods of sustained sitting (see diagram below). Be aware that vehicle vibration makes discs lose their fluid faster, so you should aim to stretch sooner than this, if you can, when travelling.

- Choose a chair with arm supports.
  Studies show that resting on your
  forearms significantly reduces lower
  back compression.

Backless kneeling chairs

The sloping seat of the backless kneeling
chair creates an optimal hollowing of
the low back, and triggers engagement
of the relevant back and tummy muscles,
but trying to use one of these too early in
the rehabilitation process – when you are
likely to over-use your back muscles, which
you are already having trouble 'switching
off' – is likely to set you back.

If you have one, start by using it for short
periods only, allowing your back muscles to
become accustomed to the increased
activity. Care should be taken if you have
knee or ankle problems, because these chairs
put weight on bent knee joints and put
pressure on the front of the ankles. Some

people find this position uncomfortable to maintain for any length of time, so you really need to visit a showroom where you can 'test drive' one of these chairs before buying.

Some of the cheaper kneeling chairs are short on padding for the kneeler bar, and also lack height and angle adjustment. Steer clear of these if at all possible.

In the longer term, and to help prevent the back problems that go with sedentary occupations, the kneeling chair can be really useful, but it's probably best to 'mix and match'. In the early days of your recovery, spending part of the working day on a conventional chair is important, as your back has to be able to cope with standard chairs and sitting postures. When using any chair it's important to have a pillow properly positioned in the lumbar hollow because it's true that one bad chair experience can set you right back. If the chair is really monstrously uncomfortable, it is better to sacrifice your pride and stuff a handbag or rolled-up jacket behind the small of your back so you can sit back and relax! (See page 153 for details of where to purchase a kneeling chair.)

Squatting

Squatting is the spine's natural decompressor, particularly if you pull your tummy in and hump out your lower back. Freestanding squatting (with your elbows on your knees) naturally recruits all your lower muscles, including your pelvic floor, but it is harder to balance. Holding on to a solid object, like the side of the bath, and leaning back as you squat adds an element of stretch right up through your spine to your chest and upper back, which helps with the releasing process through your body.

Squatting is a wonderful antidote to the compression caused by sitting and standing where the segments at the base of the spine bunch together, like one end of an elongated concertina. You should use a BackBlock (see page 73) in the evening to pull the spinal segments apart and allow the parched lower discs to suck in fluid, but you can squat through the day much more readily. Squatting opens the back of the spinal segments more and is a very dynamic way of stimulating the discs.

Sometimes, you can feel an almost irresistible desire to squat, say if you are standing in a slow-moving queue, and you shouldn't hesitate to obey the body's signals. You should also aim to squat occasionally during high-impact sport or playing golf – when it is an ideal way to line up the ball. But whatever you are doing, you should also be squatting several times a day at regular intervals.

The knees often complain at first, and if you have serious knee problems you may not be able to squat all the way down. However, most knees soon learn to love the stretch, so give them a chance to get there.

How to squat properly

1. Stand with your feet together and hold on to something secure, such as the ledge of the sink, or a gate-post.

2. Keep your feet together and your heels on the ground. Bend your knees fully and open them as wide apart as you can as you go down.

3. Squat low, keeping your head down as low as you can, rounding your spine from the base of your skull to your bottom.

4. Lean back and also feel the pull through the side of your chest wall into your armpits.

Stretch your spine by pulling your tummy in and trying to elongate your spine from the base down, to get your bottom closer to the floor.

5. In this position suck your tummy in, round out your low back even more, and gently bounce your bottom closer to the floor. You can almost feel your spine lengthening as you pull your tummy in.

6. Continue for about 30 seconds, then stand up by keeping your tummy in and pushing up through your thighs. Repeat twice.

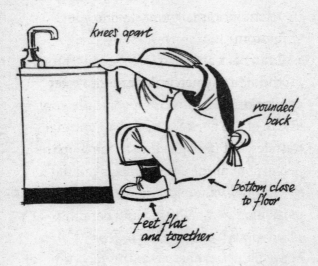

knees apart

rounded back

bottom close to floor

feet flat and together

The pelvic floor

The pelvic floor muscles form a sort of hammock at the base of the pelvis, providing support for the pelvic organs and abdominal contents.

A strong pelvic floor acts as an effective retaining wall across the floor of the trunk, assisting the tummy in raising the pressure in your abdominal cavity to brace and support the lumbar vertebrae.

Strength of the pelvic floor tends to get overlooked. It seems that people are very aware of the need for strong abdominal muscles, but in neglecting to draw up the pelvic floor at the same time as pulling in the tummy, valuable support is lost – particularly when lifting and bending.

Pelvic floor weakness is extremely common and can be caused by a variety of factors including weight gain, natural ageing, hormonal changes, pregnancy and childbirth, and pelvic surgery (particularly in men). However, the pelvic floor can also be stretched and weakened by fanatical sit-ups or crunches through the powerful bearing down forces these exercises create. You will see in the BackBlock regime in Chapter Four that 'reverse curl-ups' (exercise 3) are used to provide abdominal strength and core stability instead of old-fashioned sit-ups.

The pelvic floor exercises are the same for men and women, but before you start you must first isolate the muscles around the back passage (anus) and the front passage (urethra).

How to isolate the pelvic floor muscles

Lie down comfortably, and make sure your tummy and buttock muscles are relaxed. Now, tighten the muscles around your front and back passage, squeezing tight and drawing upwards inside at the same time. Do your best to keep all your other muscles relaxed, and don't hold your breath. As soon as you feel you have isolated the right muscles, let them relax again. It may take some time to feel these muscles working, so do be patient. As soon as you can feel those muscles switching on and off, you can begin the strengthening.

Exercise 1

1. Tighten the muscles around back and front passages while keeping all the other muscles relaxed.
2. Hold the contraction for 5 seconds, squeezing as forcefully as possible.
3. Release the contraction completely for 5–10 seconds.
4. Repeat the exercise up to 10 times per session.
5. Repeat each session up to 6 times a day.

Exercise 2

1. Follow exercise 1 by practising quick contractions.

2. Draw up and hold for just one second, then relax fully and almost immediately draw up again.

3. Aim for 10 quick contractions, one after the other.

Bending and lifting

Bending is good for you, but staying bent over for long periods is not. Dynamic bending helps circulate fluid through the discs, which keeps backs healthy. Natural bending means going down and up quickly, using all your muscles at the same time – tummy, back, buttocks and legs. Automatically, it also brings in the all-important deep spinal muscles, which control the individual spinal segments and help keep everything in place.

How to bend properly

1. Pre-hump your back prior to bending by pulling your navel in hard, and tightening the muscles of your bottom and pelvic floor. Keep these groups tight throughout the bend.
2. Keeping your knees slightly bent as you go down will help you round your back.

3. To straighten up, keep the muscles of your tummy and bottom as clenched as possible, roll your pelvis back and unfurl segment by segment up through your spine, with your head coming up last.

> *Hold everything in as you bend down and come up again normally and quickly.*

Lifting is just weighted bending, and backs are designed to lift. The action of lowering and raising the top-heavy column as you lift requires additional coordinated control of back trunk and leg muscles, and safe lifting necessitates making your back as secure as possible. However, if you haven't lifted for years, it's easy to see how your back can react by becoming stuck in a cycle of soreness as soon as you try. Using your back naturally is important to keep it healthy, and

all recovering backs need to start bending –
and eventually lifting – to recover fully.
At first, the lifting should be nothing more
than the weight of a pair of shoes, but
eventually, you can progress to shopping
bags heavy enough to nearly break the bag!
Remember, all backs will not be fully
rehabilitated until they are lifting 'normal
everyday things' again. Bracing the spine
from the front with maximum tummy
strength is the main clue to safe lifting.

How to lift properly

1. Your spinal segments are more stable
   when the discs are maximally
   pressurised, and this is achieved when
   you pre-hump your lower back. So, just
   as with bending, you need to really pull
   in your tummy muscles, the muscles of
   your bottom and the pelvic floor, and
   forcibly round out your lower back to
   keep all the lumbar segments secure
   throughout the lift.

2. Your legs need to work strongly when you lift. You do this by bending your knees as you bend your back, which allows the powerful front thigh muscles to help.

3. Know the weight of the object in advance of the lift, and if you are concerned it is too heavy, it probably is!

4. Make sure you get a secure grip on the object to be lifted, and keep it close in to your body.

5. For bigger, unwieldy objects, try to ensure you have adequate space around the object to be lifted – remove obstacles in your path, and plan your route.

6. If you are lifting a heavier weight, squat down with your feet apart (a nice wide base will make you more stable), bending your knees and hips as much as you need.

7. When coming up, make sure your tummy and the muscles of your bottom are really tight, roll your pelvis back and

straighten your back and legs at the same time, as quickly as possible.

When you are learning to lift again, expect the back to be sore afterwards. You cannot go at it too hard, and always limit yourself to a couple of times a day at first (otherwise your back will lurch back into crisis). In the early days, you might bend to pick up your child's school bag, say, but you should counter this straight away by doing the 'spinal appeasing' exercises (see pages 80–98) to calm the back down again. For the first few weeks, you *must always* settle your back like this whenever you have lifted. Although it may take up time in your day, it is the best way to ensure your back doesn't ache and become sore as it gets accustomed to the new rules.

FOUR

THE MAIN SELF-TREATMENT EXERCISES

Although all five stages of spinal breakdown seem radically different, regardless of which stage most accurately fits your particular back condition, the key to successful treatment is addressing the painful tightness (and scarring) of a spinal link and drawing water through its drier disc. This is done through regular, daily exercises directed at your problem level. This section deals with the vitally important exercise routine to help you un-jam your back, make the outer disc wall more stretchable, and improve disc nutrition.

Read all the exercises through before starting, as not every exercise is suitable for your back trouble.

The first three exercises in this section form the core of the BackBlock regime. These exercises work together to stretch and strengthen your lumbar spine, to improve the fluid exchange through your lumbar discs, relax tight muscles and develop a girdle of muscle support to help you protect your back.

Some may find exercise 4, 'legs passing', easier or more appropriate than exercise 3, 'reverse curls', but read the introduction and 'how to do' sections carefully before trying either.

Start by aiming to complete the regime (exercises 1–3) twice, increasing to three times as you feel able.

Exercise 1: The BackBlock

A BackBlock is a brick-shaped block made of high-density foam, wood or plastic. BackBlocks come with instructions that must be strictly followed. See page 153 for details of how to purchase the Sarah Key BackBlocks.

Instead of a BackBlock you can use a 5cm stack of books. But the advantage of the Block is that the 'how to' instructions are glued to it and its height can easily be varied by turning the block on its side and even on its end (see page 78). You can also use a brick-sized yoga block, available at most good sports shops, but make sure you carefully follow the instructions spelled out below. Also make sure it is wide enough to support you comfortably when positioned under your sacrum.

Regular use of a BackBlock forms the core of your spinal decompression regime. It provides a safe and effective way of opening and closing the lumbar segments, inducing fluid movement through the discs, and stretching the outer disc wall to make it more compliant and comfortable to stretch. Using the BackBlock helps counter the day-long compressive forces of standing and sitting, and the dramatic on–off pressure changes improve disc cellular activity and metabolic vigour.

How to use the BackBlock properly

1. Lie on the floor on your back with your knees bent.
2. Gently lift your bottom by rounding your low back and rolling up your spine, coming off the floor one vertebra at a time.
3. Slide the BackBlock under your sacrum (the hard flat bone at the base of your

spine), making sure it is positioned low down.

4. Pull your tummy in hard to protect your back, straighten each leg, one at a time, by pushing your heel out slowly along the floor. Make sure *not to lift* each leg as you straighten it!

5. Relax, and let your body go heavy as you lie there.

When you are satisfied the BackBlock is in the correct position (you often have to move it about a bit until it feels comfortable, and remember, *where it feels comfortable is where it should be!*), completely let everything go, and relax on the Block.

As you drape yourself back over the BackBlock, relax every muscle in your body.

If you feel inclined, take your arms above your head and let them flop back on the floor behind you. Otherwise, leave your arms by your sides and let them roll out, with your palms facing the ceiling.

After 60 seconds (or less, if it becomes really uncomfortable) pull your tummy in hard, bend one knee at a time as you slide your heel up the floor to your bottom, and lift off the Block as you slide it away. It almost always hurts to raise your bottom off the Block, but don't panic! Any discomfort should pass within a few seconds, and then you will continue to 'ease' your back by going into the following exercise.

The BackBlock followed by exercise 2 'knees rocking' and exercise 3 'reverse curl-ups' form the three important steps of the BackBlock regime. Failing to follow the BackBlock with these two exercises almost always leads to increased back soreness!

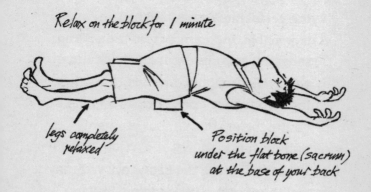

Relax on the block for 1 minute

legs completely
relaxed

Position block
under the flat bone (sacrum)
at the base of your back

Trouble-shooting for the BackBlock

- Don't use the BackBlock if your back is
  very painful or rigid with muscle spasm.
  You must use your instincts here and
  wait for any severe discomfort to subside
  before taking to it again. This could
  mean leaving off it for 7 to 10 days and
  doing the full 'spinal appeasing' regime
  (see exercises 2–5 below) in the interim.

- Try to relax as much as possible when on
  the Block. Let the muscles of your bottom
  relax and feel your legs roll out.
  Remember, the greater the degree of
  relaxation, the greater the separation of

the vertebrae. You should feel an 'agreeable discomfort' from the pulling sensation through your low back and across the front of your hips. Don't fight it; let your body open out and feel the gentle tug of your lumbar segments pulling apart.

- When first using the BackBlock you may feel the stretch a little too much. For several weeks, if necessary, you can use a flatter object (say a book) before working up to the lowest height of the Block.

- As your back starts to feel easier, you may progress to using the BackBlock on its middle side and eventually up-ended (although it can take years to get to this stage). *The main thing is to relax and not be in too much of a hurry* to move on to the next stage. No matter how advanced you are, you should always start each session with the Block on its flattest side. Although the extra height provides more effective decompression, it is harder to relax, and being too gung-ho can leave the back stirred up.

- Make sure you pass through the three steps of the BackBlock routine with no sense of urgency; one step leading into the next in a continuum of languid, flowing movement. Don't try too hard and don't allow your movements to become hasty or jerky. Often, slowing down is part of the healing process!

- Never extend the length of time you are on the Block. More is not better. Remember, you are looking for 'pressure changes' over a short period, and three goes of one minute (with its following steps 2 and 3) is far more effective than one long three-minute session.

- Never position the Block under your lumbar vertebrae; it must be lower down under your sacrum to get the benefit of the stretch and separation of those lower segments.

Exercise 2: Knees rocking

This is such an important exercise, and really comes into its own if you have just hurt your back. Its gentle pumping action softens the clench of muscles in spasm, and helps evacuate the swelling of fluid trapped, both within the discs and around the facet joints. In the longer term, rocking your knees also has a positive therapeutic effect. It pulls in tide after tide of fluids through the back wall of the discs, improving vascular exchange, and giving this hard-working part of the disc first use of the nutrients coming in, which helps the repair of fibre damage and scarring.

Always go straight into this exercise on coming off the BackBlock, because it will relieve the momentary discomfort you may feel when lifting your bottom off the Block. Ease into it gently, quietly rocking for as long as it takes for your back to feel comfortable again. This may take a couple of minutes. If your back is really screaming, this may be the only exercise you can do. Follow the instructions below, but rest your lower legs on pillows in between times.

As soon as the severe pain has subsided, add exercise 3 or 4 to activate your tummy muscles; then bring in exercise 5 to help switch off spasm and improve muscle coordination. Exercises 2–5 constitute your very important 'spinal appeasing' regime – so-called because it consists of the exercises best suited to relieve and pacify a back in crisis to relieve pain and get you back on track with progress.

How to do 'knees rocking' properly

1. Lie on your back on a folded towel on a carpeted floor.
2. Tighten your tummy muscles as you bring first the right knee up to your chest, holding it with your right hand, then the other knee.

3. If possible, cross your ankles and spread your knees wide (this makes the legs less unwieldy).

4. Gently rock your knees backwards and forwards with your head relaxed on the floor. Get into a rhythm of small and subtle movements, which should bring a sense of muscles relaxing and the back softening as it opens up.

5. You may alternate between rocking back and forth with side to side and small circles, first clockwise then anti-clockwise, going up and down the spine. These small movements can help you get to know your back, to identify the stiff patches. By staying on them and gently

Don't be too gung-ho with this exercise. Think of pumping, rather than stretching, and let your head float away.

oscillating over them, you will feel the stiffness 'melt' and the discomfort fade. See it rather like polishing rust off a metal object; making the metal smooth and shiny again.

6. Take your time with this, oscillating your knees gently at about one cycle per second, pausing whenever you like, but you can continue for up to 5 minutes. For a newly injured back, repeat every 2 hours.

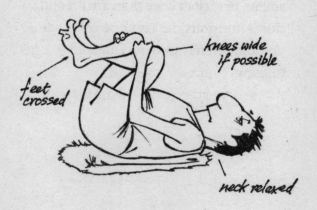

knees wide if possible

feet crossed

neck relaxed

Trouble-shooting 'knees rocking'

- Never lie on the BackBlock while carrying out the knees rocking exercise.
- Keep your tummy muscles relaxed when you are rocking your knees and leave your head resting on the floor.
- The smaller the movement and the gentler you are with this exercise, the more your spine will relax. Remember, less is more!
- It can be tempting to use a big rocking action, but try to keep it a smooth and subtle 'local' action. Think of gently pumping rather than pulling and tugging.

Exercise 3: Reverse curl-ups

This is the ideal way to strengthen weak tummy muscles, but some people find exercise 4, 'legs passing', easier to do. Reverse curl-ups strengthen the lower abdominal muscles, particularly below navel level, which are more directly responsible for supporting the low spinal segments. Effective control from the lower abdominals (lower tummy muscles) is vitally important in protecting your back during bending and lifting. While conventional sit-ups can cause shearing strain across the lumbar segments, reverse curl-ups are completely safe.

How to do 'reverse curl-ups' properly

1. Lie on your back on a carpeted floor with your fingers interlaced behind your head.
2. Pull in your tummy muscles and draw one knee at a time to your chest. Cross your ankles and open your knees as wide as possible.

3. Without jerking, round your lower back as you lift your bottom off the floor, tightening and drawing up the pelvic floor at the same time.

4. Move your knees towards your chin and down again, mainly through the action of bending and unbending your lower back, rather than just the hips. This action may be difficult and slightly ungainly at first, but do persevere.

5. Do not let your thighs drop beyond the vertical on the way down, as this will strain your back.

6. Repeat 15 times, making sure you go up and down at the same speed.

Gently rock your knees back and forth at the same speed, remembering to tighten the pelvic floor as your back rounds and your knees draw up towards your chin.

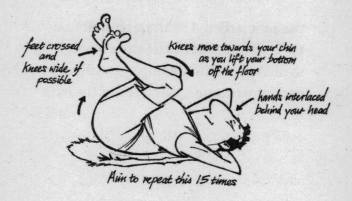

feet crossed and knees wide if possible

knees move towards your chin as you lift your bottom off the floor

hands interlaced behind your head

Aim to repeat this 15 times

Trouble-shooting 'reverse curl-ups'

- If you have a neck problem, you might find it better to place your palms upwards on your forehead. This minimises any strain to your neck caused by the abdominal effort.

- You may feel that your roll-up action is very modest and your low back barely bends, but that's fine. Try not to cheat by throwing your feet over your head with a knee-straightening action, which achieves only minimal rounding of your lumbar spine. Your thighs should remain at the same angle to your chest and all the action should be through your low back; as you go up, there should be a shrinking and tightening at the front and rounding and stretching at the back.

Exercise 4: Legs passing

This is often viewed as an easier version of exercise 3, 'reverse curl-ups', but this varies from person to person. It requires concentration to move the legs fluently past one another without wobbling or arching the back, and is an effective exercise for tricking the tummy muscles into working again after back injury. It is also a marvellous way of getting the lower back moving, and the hips swinging more freely during walking.

Keep your abdominal muscles fully switched on so that your low back remains pressed into the floor, and your legs move slowly and under control.

How to do 'legs passing' properly

1. Lie on your back on a carpeted floor with your fingers interlaced behind your head (only if you are having difficulty initially should you leave your arms beside you as shown in the diagram). Tighten your tummy muscles as hard as possible, rolling your pelvis back to press your low back into the floor.

2. Bring your left knee towards your left armpit with the knee fully bent, making sure that your tummy muscles remain rigorously switched on all the time. As you start returning your left leg to the floor, begin lifting the right leg so that the legs pass one another in mid-air in the middle part of range.

3. The heel of your returning foot should just skim the floor, close to your bottom, before making the return journey towards your armpit. Do not let the returning foot rest on the floor between excursions, and do not straighten either knee during the exercise.

4. Continue for 60 seconds, moving the legs slowly with rhythm and control.

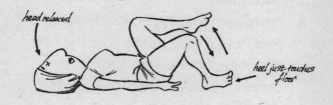

head relaxed

heel just touches floor

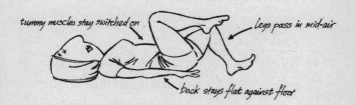

tummy muscles stay switched on

legs pass in mid-air

back stays flat against floor

Trouble-shooting 'legs passing'

● The most common mistake with this exercise is straightening out the descending leg as if 'cycling in mid-air'. Lowering a straight leg can cause discomfort and puts a *huge* strain on the lower back.

- Don't allow your concentration to lapse and your low back to come up, away from the floor, as this may also cause discomfort.
- Try to keep your upper body relaxed, your head resting on the floor and your neck long. If this proves difficult, try clasping your hands together and resting them under your chin or on the front of your forehead, which can act as a gentle reminder to keep your head down and your neck long.
- Pull up through your pelvic floor for the whole time your abdominal muscles are engaged, but don't hold your breath.
- Be sure to make a full excursion with both legs; up as high as you can towards the armpit and down the full journey to the floor, just brushing the floor with the heel of your foot before you return. Try not to cheat and shorten the descent by touching the floor with your toe only.

But do not let the foot rest on the floor, either, making it far too easy to lift the other leg. Make sure the legs do pass in mid-air.

- While doing this exercise, make a mental note of the degree to which your tummy muscles are switched on, and try to replicate it exactly while walking; girding yourself in and up, and moving 'lightly' forward as you swing your hips and walk freely. Pulling in your tummy as you walk helps enormously in improving posture and supporting your back.

Exercise 5: Spinal rolling

At first glance, this exercise seems absurdly easy but in fact it is highly sophisticated. Tipping back and forth along your spine requires coordinated control of muscles both back and front, which is important when your back is in alarm; when your back muscles won't switch off and your tummy muscles won't switch on! The rolling action also helps break up the armour-plated brittleness of your low back, loosening the individual segments from the grip of over-active back muscles.

A fluent rolling action can take a while to coordinate, and this can be discouraging. But as you get more proficient, you can fine-tune the excursions so that eventually you are pivoting only on the problem spinal link(s). Initially, this can be difficult because the tendency will be to scoot over the stiff patches, like 'kerthumping' over a square wheel. Remember, it is harder to do this exercise finely than it is to rock back and forth with gay abandon. With time, and experimenting with the leverage of your legs, by bending or straightening the knees, you will also be able to isolate other problem levels higher up your spine.

How to do 'spinal rolling' properly

1. Lying on a yoga mat or similar padded surface on the floor, gather your legs up one at a time and clasp your hands around (or behind) your knees while rounding your back and tucking your chin to chest.
2. Gently roll back and forth along your spine, pausing to pivot on the painful segments.
3. Continue for 15 to 30 seconds, continuing to pay most attention to the flatter patches in your spine.
4. Rest by releasing your legs one at a time, with your tummy muscles switched on.

Keep your knees bent and feet on the floor, and rest for 1 minute then resume the rocking as before.

5. Having your legs quite long (rather than knees bunched up) changes the leverage and makes it easier to spend time down the lower end of your spine where the spinal links are more needy.

6. Repeat up to three times.

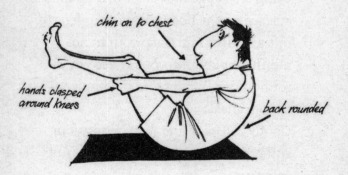

chin on to chest

hands clasped around knees

back rounded

Trouble-shooting 'spinal rolling'

- It's easy to bruise your spine by over-vigorous rolling on a hard floor, so make sure you are using a sufficiently padded surface.

Make the back and forth movement as fluent as possible, trying not to jerk your neck. Do not come up to sitting on your bottom.

- The most common mistake here is coming up to sit on your bottom each time you roll down the spine. This will interrupt the rhythm and add unwanted compression when you are trying to give your low back a breather from these forces.
- It is unimportant whether you hold your hands capped over each knee, your fingers interlaced behind, or whether you hold the backs of your thighs. It all seems to depend on how strong you are in the tummy and how heavy your upper body is.

- Try not to jerk your neck to tip you forward. Make the back and forth journeys as streamlined as possible, without jarring as you change direction.
- Keep breathing normally as you rock, and try to relax your chin on to your chest. Forcing your chin down will alter your breathing and strain your neck.

Exercise 6: Pelvic bridging

Again, this exercise seems deceptively easy, but apart from making it easier to move your body around in bed, it is an important strengthener of the key muscle groups providing bending power to your back. When backs are disabled by pain, they lose the ability to control the individual segments. As a result, the back moves as a rigid mass, and bending becomes precarious. The well-meaning but erroneous instruction to 'keep the back straight and bend the knees' makes matters worse. This exercise is the safest way to re-learn bending from the basics.

Both your deep abdominal and spinal muscles, working together as you roll up and down the spine, create a sort of undulating wave-like action through the back which, after years of neglect, may be difficult to restore. This gentle, controlled movement of individual spinal segments helps to break up the rod-like rigidity of a spine which has become unaccustomed to movement. It improves coordinated interplay between dominant and long-forgotten muscles, while at the same time improving the fluid flow through the discs.

How to do 'pelvic bridging' properly

1. Lie on your back on the floor with your knees bent and feet placed as close as possible to your bottom. Rest your arms by your side, or better still, over your head on the floor, fingers interlaced and palms turned away.
2. Pre-hump your lower back by clenching your bottom and pulling in your tummy hard.
3. Roll up your spine segment by segment until your body forms a straight line between shoulders, hips and knees to make a bridge.
4. Keep your knees pinned together to switch on the muscles of your bottom.

5   Hold the position for 15 seconds, then begin the return journey by sucking your tummy in and rolling down your spine segment by segment, paying particular attention to the stiff patches, until the very base of your spine rests on the floor.

6.   Repeat three times.

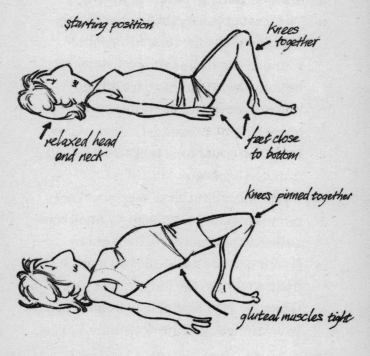

starting position

knees together

relaxed head and neck

feet close to bottom

knees pinned together

gluteal muscles tight

As you lift your bottom off the floor, try to roll up your spine, vertebra by vertebra, to the base of your neck.

Trouble-shooting 'pelvic bridging'

- The most obvious problem here is the inability to get the back sufficiently rounded. Instead, as you go to lift your bottom, the whole low back lifts en masse like a plank. Pre-humping the lower back by pressing it into the floor helps you roll around it like a wheel, from the base up.
- If you find it difficult to keep your knees pinned together, try holding a small book there for the duration of the exercise.
- If your muscles are weak, you may be unable to make the line straight. Don't worry. Do your best and, with practice, your strength will improve quite quickly.

Exercise 7: Toe touches

This exercise both stretches and strengthens as it carefully introduces the spine to 'natural bending'. Bending forward stretches and thins the facet joint capsules and the backs of the discs, improving disc hydration and repair. Controlled unfurling from bent to upright is an important muscle strengthener.

The key with this exercise is *control*. The careful going down and the more dynamically active unfurling back to upright, vertebra by vertebra, improves the strength and responsiveness of the deep back muscles and is vitally important for thorough back rehabilitation. Don't be afraid of toe touching, but read the instructions carefully and follow them to the letter to ensure it is safe and effective (see 'Bending and lifting' on page 63 for more information). Remember that initially you may need to do a lot of 'spinal appeasing' (see exercises 2–5 on pages 80–98) after first starting this exercise. Don't worry. This is absolutely normal.

How to do 'toe touches' properly

1. Stand tall with feet about 15cm apart.
2. Tighten your bottom, pull up your pelvic floor, and pull in your tummy, pre-humping the low back to 'prime' your discs in preparation for leaving the safety of vertical.
3. Unlock your knees slightly to take the tension off your hamstrings. With tummy pulled in, bring your chin to chest and bend forward by rolling from the top of the spine down, all the time the tummy held in like a greyhound.
4. At the bottom, try a few tiny bounces to increase the spinal stretch, remembering to keep your knees bent and tummy pulled in. Let your head and arms dangle free. Relax your neck, and feel as if your hair could sweep the floor.

5. Prepare for the return journey by re-clenching tummy, pelvic floor and bottom to tip the pelvis back, and unfurl to vertical cog by cog, head coming up last.

6. Repeat twice.

7. Beginners must then lie down on a soft surface and appease the spine (see exercises 2–5) after doing this exercise.

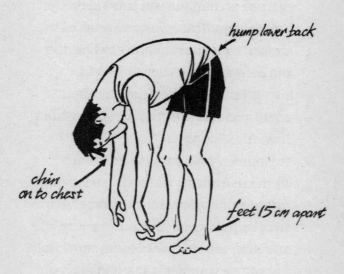

hump lower back

chin
on to chest

feet 15 cm apart

Bend forward with everything pulled in and dangle for a moment before coming up, one vertebra at a time.

Trouble-shooting 'toe touches'

- The most common mistake with this exercise is thinking you must keep the legs straight. This is not required, as the hamstring tension rolls the pelvis back and increases low back tightness.
- If your back feels weak (and it often does!), you can use your hands to walk down the thighs.
- Remember, your back is particularly vulnerable during the early part of bend, so it is vitally important to prime your discs by pulling in your tummy and rounding the low back before starting.
- Do not use your arms again to push up from the bend, as your spine needs the

strength training. Make sure to maintain the strong clench of the abdomen and buttocks all the way up.

- Take care not to switch over to using the long cable muscles halfway up, which sees the head coming up first as the upper back jack-knifes into arched extension.

- Make sure you keep a careful unfurling action going all the way to the top, head coming up last.

- This exercise is easy to over-do, which will make the back sore and even bring on long-forgotten leg pain. Make sure you do *a couple of sessions of two or three bends per day only.* Any more will set you back!

Exercise 8: Floor twists

This is a fairly advanced exercise, so be cautious when adding it to your regime. The twisting action stretches the tough diagonal mesh of the disc walls and improves vertical stretch through the low back. When you start to include this exercise, always do it before the BackBlock and you will feel a greater sense of letting go and distraction of the spinal segments. The 'floor twists' also open up the facet joints lying along the top side of your body. The same stretch also helps free up spinal nerves, if they have become tethered where they exit the spinal canal. Sometimes, the traction on the nerve root temporarily stirs up leg pain, but that is no reason to stop doing it. It simply means that you have to follow each floor twisting session with the appeasing exercises 2–5 to ease the newly irritated local soft tissues.

How to do 'floor twists' properly

1. Lie on your back and stretch your arms out from your sides on the floor at shoulder level, palms facing down.

2. Pulling your tummy in hard, lift one knee, then the other, high on to your chest, knees together.

3. Keeping knees pinned together and your tummy pulled in, let both legs fall over to the right, right leg on the floor and the left on top, with both thighs parallel and together.

4. Trying to keep your hands on the floor and your knees high, straighten the top (left) leg and attempt to take hold of this foot with the right hand.

As you hold your foot, try to let the upper body relax and the back shoulder lie back flatter on the floor.

5. Hold this stretch for 30 seconds, giving tiny bounces by pulling on the toes.

6. At the same time, try to twist your upper body back so the back of your chest is lying flatter against the floor.

7. To release, let the foot go and, bending both knees, sweep your pinned-together thighs over your abdomen to the other side. Repeat to the other side.

8. If you are much more restricted to one side (that's to say, if you find your legs won't go as freely to one side, or there is a big difference in how far you can bring them up), repeat the stretch 4 times more to the stiffer side.

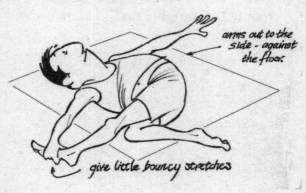

arms out to the side - against the floor.

give little bouncy stretches

Trouble-shooting 'floor twists'

- The main problem with this exercise is the temptation to bend the uppermost knee to make it possible to reach the toes.

- More effective traction is exerted on tethered nerve roots by keeping the leg straight at the knee and holding further up, say behind the calf or the knee. This will also mean that the leg does not come up as high towards the shoulder on the floor.

- If possible, try to gently draw the foot even higher up the floor, feeling the increase in stretch through the leg. It should be a 'sweet pain' along the leg as the nerve is pulled.

- Ensuring your tummy muscles stay tightly pulled in as you let your knees fall to the side will help to protect your back as you twist.

- Do the same thing as you return your knees to your chest, attempting as much as you can to use your tummy muscles (the obliques) rather than pushing through your arms.

- Try to keep the hand behind you pressed flat to the floor with the palm facing down. Tight chest and pectoral muscles will make this arm want to float off the floor.

Exercise 9: Child pose

This is the safest and most unthreatening way to introduce bending, and is especially useful for people who have kept their back straight for years. It opens up the back of the segments, stretching tight disc walls and facet joints. It is an excellent antidote to the day-long compression caused by standing and sitting, and is a calming stretch at the end of your exercise routine.

How to do 'child pose' properly

1. Kneel on the floor with feet together and the upper surface of your feet flat against the floor.
2. Separate your knees, sit your bottom back on your heels and lower your upper body towards the floor, as far as possible nestling your belly down between your thighs.
3. Flatten out as much as possible, stretching your arms in front along the floor.

4. Pull in your tummy muscles, rounding your low back and attempting to stretch your tailbone towards the floor. You should feel an agreeable pull as your spine elongates.

5. Hold the stretch for 1 minute, staying as relaxed as you can and breathing normally.

6. There is no need to repeat this stretch at the end of your exercise routine, but feel free to carry out the 'child pose' whenever you feel the need to stretch out your low back. You will find that making the effort to get to the floor is always worthwhile.

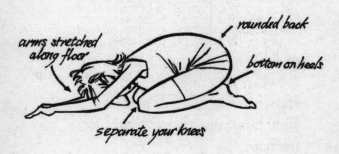

arms stretched along floor

rounded back

bottom on heels

separate your knees

Try to get as flat to the floor as possible, nestling your belly down between the knees. Initially, it may be hard on the knees and feet.

Trouble-shooting 'child pose'

- Keep your neck muscles relaxed and your head down to the floor as you stretch. This will help you round your back and make the most of the lengthening through your spine.
- It is not uncommon for knees to 'complain' when you first start this exercise. However, most people find that after a day or two, the knee stiffness melts away, leaving the knees feeling much freer.
- If knee discomfort persists, it might help to pop a pillow over your calves to rest your thighs on. This reduces the bend through your knee joints.

- If your ankles are stiff, sitting back on your heels can be problematic and uncomfortable. In such cases, a small folded towel placed under the feet can make all the difference.

Exercise 10: Cobra

This is an advanced exercise. The weighted backward arching here stretches the front of the spine and hips, as it lengthens muscles and other soft tissues habitually shortened by excessive hours of crumpled sitting. Although the action appears similar to the passive arching of using the BackBlock, the dynamics are entirely different. By pushing up from the prone position through the hands, the bone-against-bone facet joints at the back of the spine override or compress, which in some instances can aggravate a low back problem, especially if it is done too early, or in the acute stage of rehabilitation, when the back is still easily irritated and can be stirred up by relatively minor increases in exercise or activity. Even later on, it is always wise to follow 'the cobra' with appeasing exercises 2–5, but be prepared to stop completely if it triggers pain that persists the next day.

> *Make sure your hands do not creep forward on the floor or your elbows bend as this will reduce the efficacy of this stretch.*

In the later, more chronic, stages of rehabilitation, when the problem segment is not too irritable, the short-term compression of the joint surfaces, caused by the facet joints overriding, helps stimulate regeneration of the mother-of-pearl cartilage buffer that covers the bone.

Also, the on–off pressure changes can be an effective way of 'milking' a chronically engorged facet joint capsule. This is particularly effective when followed by exercise 9 'child pose' (see page 113).

How to do 'cobra' properly

1. Lie face down on the floor with your hands palm down on the floor beneath your shoulders.

2. Push your upper trunk off the floor by pushing through your arms and straightening the elbows.

3. Your aim is to straighten your elbows fully while keeping your pelvis against the floor. This may take time, but don't be tempted to slide your arms forward to make it easier. Instead, let your pelvis lift off the floor.

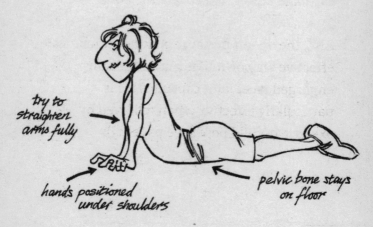

try to straighten arms fully

hands positioned under shoulders

pelvic bone stays on floor

4. Keep your neck long, and don't let your shoulders hunch up around your ears.

5. Hold this position for 30 seconds, trying to let the spine relax and drop down into a deeper saddle, as your pubic bone at the front nears the floor.

6. Come down by bending your elbows until you are lying flat. Turn your face to the side (it makes breathing easier!), and rest for 15 seconds.

7. Repeat 3 times, turning your head to alternate sides to rest.

Exercise 11: Child pose to cobra

This composite exercise is quite an advanced progression and not suitable for everyone. It takes your spine to the limits of range in both directions, which stimulates the discs and facet joint cartilage as it helps to improve muscle coordination. You may find in the early days of your back being in alarm that it takes a long time after pushing back from 'cobra' for your bottom to sink down on your heels and relax into 'child pose'. You may feel a painful guarding in the muscles across the low back, but don't worry. As things improve, they let go more quickly and your bottom settles less painfully at the end of each return journey from 'cobra'.

How to do 'child pose to cobra' properly

1. From 'child pose' position, exercise 9, get ready for lifting your bottom off your heels by tightening your tummy and humping your lower back. Sliding both

hands palm-down along the floor, take your weight forward on to your hands and knees and then further forward to just on your hands, stopping when your shoulders are directly over your hands. Allow your pelvis to sink through towards the floor.

2. Keep your elbows straight and your neck long.

3. Try to allow your muscles to relax, and hang there for 30 seconds.

4. Revert to 'child pose' by pulling in your tummy, humping your back and pushing your bottom back to your heels.

You will need to pull your tummy in hard to lift your pelvis off the floor, and push back with your sitting bones to get your bottom on your heels.

5. Remain in this position for 30 seconds and then repeat the process as above.
6. Aim to go back and forth 4 or 5 times in total, easing your pelvis closer to the floor each time.

Trouble-shooting 'child pose' to 'cobra'

- In coming out of the 'cobra', it is easy for your back to lock up painfully as you lift your pelvis from the floor and push your bottom back towards the heels. Being aware in advance makes it easier to make the transition from one position to the other but, even so, take the time to keep it steady and controlled.
- When pushing your bottom towards the heels, try to get a sense of the spine elongating as you attempt to push your sitting bones through the seat of your pants. This will better recruit your low abdominal muscles, making your low back better protected.

- Be patient with this exercise. It may take some time for your low back to be able to relax at both ends – deep into the hollow of 'cobra' and nestling the bottom down to the heels.

FIVE

DO'S AND DON'TS

Desk work

- Do ensure desk height, computer set-up and lighting are all adjusted to create a more comfortable working environment. Office workers should be offered an ergonomic assessment of their work station to help achieve optimal conditions. If you haven't been offered this service, you should ask for it.

- If you work from home, check that your chair and desk height allow you to sit comfortably, with adequate clearance between your thighs and the underside of the desk. Your work surface should be flat and stable, and your monitor and keyboard should be positioned in front of you. Set the monitor so that the top of the casing is 5–8cm above eye level, and sit at arm's length from your monitor.

- Remove clutter from under your desk. You should have adequate leg room but be able to draw your chair as close as possible to your desk.

- Your office chair should swivel so that you don't have to twist repeatedly to reach your phone or PC.

- Remember to squat regularly throughout the day to relieve the compression through your low back. When taking your allotted breaks, take them away from your desk if possible. Try to fit in a walk at lunch time as this will help you free up stiffened joints and muscles.

- Stay hydrated. Regular visits to the water cooler (or the tap) will give you a break from sitting, and lead to more frequent visits to the bathroom, where you can hang off a wash basin to do your squats (see page 55).

- Do have regular eye tests. If you are straining to read your computer screen, that strain will refer into the muscles of your neck and back, exacerbating spasm and pain.

Exercise

- Do your back exercises every day, but don't over-exercise. Remember that often less is more. Don't be too prescriptive with your exercises and learn to 'listen' to your back.
- Do be prepared to ease off on your exercises if your back remains very sore and use the appeasing exercises (pages 80–98) to get you back on track.
- Do try to walk each day, but monitor the impact on your back, and increase your distance slowly. Wear supportive footwear and stride out, keeping your tummy drawn in and walking light, thinking of making minimal impact on the ground.
- Once your back problem is well under control, improving general fitness will bring long-term benefits to your back, and bolster your morale. Remember to use caution when embarking on any

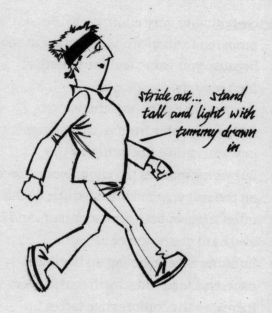

stride out... stand tall and light with tummy drawn in

new fitness regime and also remember that indiscriminate exercising can set you back.

- Yoga combines the benefits of controlled stretch and strengthening in a non-competitive, centring and calming way. However, there are many different forms of yoga ranging from extremely gentle to absurdly energetic, and teacher skill and class quality vary enormously. Be prepared to shop around. Be patient too because you won't feel the benefits immediately.

- Swimming can be a useful way to improve aerobic fitness. The movement in water can be liberating, as the buoyancy reduces the compressive forces on the spine. Avoid breaststroke, as this often triggers back and neck pain, and is also hard on the knees.

- Running is very jarring on the lower back, and road running in particular increases the compressive forces up through the lumbar spine. Brisk walking is better for your back.

- Old-fashioned 'sit-ups' or 'crunches' can be disastrous for a bad back, simply because they can easily be done badly. The lurching action, often associated with trying to achieve a high number of repetitions (we call this end-scoring) can cause serious shearing strains across the lumbar segments. It can also overwork the upper abdominals, leaving a pouchy, soft under belly below the navel. The strenuous hinging action at the hips, in combination with a poor spinal curling action, also increases compression through the low back which may trigger further spasm and joint soreness. On the other hand, 'reverse curl-ups' (see exercise 3, page 85) work the all-important lower abdominals, prevent hinging at the hips, and decompress your low back while strengthening your stomach muscles safely.

Walk tall and light with your midriff reefed in.

Gardening

- The all-important thing is to factor in enough time to run through your BackBlock regime when your gardening session is over.
- Vary your tasks so that you are never spending extended periods in one position.
- Bending is good for you, but staying bent will make your back sore. So straighten up regularly, remembering to 'pull everything in' before coming up.
- Kneel for the fiddly jobs, such as weeding or planting seedlings. Remember, too, the importance of engaging your tummy muscles as you reach forward.
- Pushing a heavily laden wheelbarrow is punishment for your back, as it causes shear on the lower segments. Don't overload the barrow and if it is really heavy, you are better off pulling it rather than pushing.

- Squat regularly (see page 55) to give your compressed discs a much-needed drink.
- Try to ensure that your gardening tools are fit for purpose. The wrong-size spade or fork can make the task much more difficult, which can be costly for your back.
- When digging, use your body weight on the spade. This is much more effective than simply using your arms.

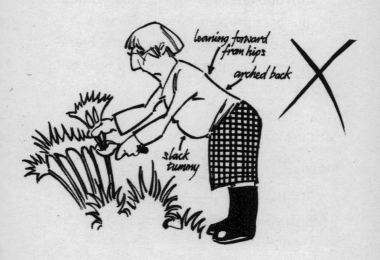

Shopping

- Lifting and carrying bags of shopping need not be detrimental to your back, but don't overload yourself, and balance the load evenly in both hands.
- Remember to prime your back in readiness for lifting, by pulling in your tummy muscles hard and rounding your low back.
- Supermarket trolleys – especially those with dubious steering – can aggravate your back problems. Try to choose a small trolley, ensure it steers well, brace with your tummy muscles and walk tall as you push.

Always pull your tummy in hard when pushing a shopping trolley or lifting shopping bags.

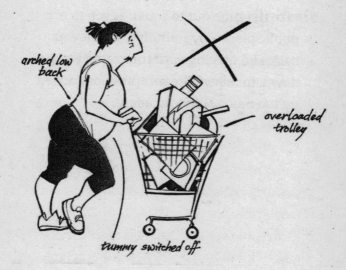

arched low back

overloaded trolley

tummy switched off

- It is better to put your shopping in the boot of the car rather than the back seat because it is easier to get at. Either way, make sure you keep your tummy braced as you reach in to heave it out.
- Most backs hate long periods of standing, or the slow shuffle of window-shopping, which should be avoided when your back is sore. If you can, and you don't feel too self-conscious, try to

take the time out to squat – even in a public place – by rounding your lower back and bracing your tummy as you go down, to relieve the compression caused by too much standing about.

SIX

FREQUENTLY ASKED QUESTIONS

Q. Why is my back so stiff when I try to get out of bed in the morning?

A. There are several possible reasons for early-morning back stiffness. Movement keeps our joints 'oiled', and worn joints tend to stiffen more quickly than pristine ones. For this reason, lack of movement during sleep can cause a slight seizing of worn joints. When we lie down, compression through our discs is relieved, and the process of rehydration begins again. Fluid is sucked into the discs overnight, so that we gain approximately 2cm in height (we lose it again during the next day as water is leached out, carrying waste products).

When the discs are full in the morning, the sensitive outer disc wall can be painfully stretched. When we get up and start moving around, muscle activity and gravitational forces start evacuating fluid again, making the back more comfortable as the tension on the wall is reduced.

Q. Is a hard mattress better for my back?

A. There is a world of difference between hard, and supportive. Your spine needs to be buoyed up by your mattress, but a really hard mattress is less likely to support the contours of your back as you sleep. Equally so, a really old mattress is unlikely to be giving you the support you need. Different beds suit different people, but a saggy mattress can never be good for your back. If you feel uncomfortable on your bed, but okay in another one, it's time you changed your bed.

If you are forced to sleep on an unsuitably hard or saggy mattress – as so often happens when travelling – try folding a large towel into a tube and wrapping that around your waist to fill the gap between your pelvis and ribcage when you are lying on your side. Pillows under your knees will help support your lumbar spine if you are lying on your back.

There are many considerations when choosing a good bed, so you have to take the time to try each one – and that means lying on them in the shop! A good mattress has sufficient thrusting support from within, so that you feel 'spring-loaded' as you turn over at night. A good mattress should also be springy and supportive when you sit down on the side of the bed. There are other issues to consider too, such as the base on which the mattress sits, and the weight (and build) of the occupant(s).

Q. Is a memory foam mattress good for my back?

A. Some people swear by a memory foam mattress, while others are decidedly unimpressed by them. Although it is true that this type of mattress provides support and ample cushioning for your back, its ability to mould to the contours of your body can make changing position much more of an effort. If you stiffen up at night and need to shift around a lot in your bed, then this type of mattress may not be suitable.

Q. Does it matter what sort of shoes I wear?

A. Yes, it does but in many instances, the shock absorption qualities of the shoe are more important than the height of the heel. The main thing is that your shoes should be both supportive and cushioning when you walk. Pavements are unforgiving and unnaturally jarring, so providing a cushioned sole between your foot and hard surfaces makes the world of difference to absorbing impact.

Wearing cushioning insoles can help minimise the jarring of unyielding heels. Tottering along on high heels alters your centre of gravity, and makes you engage all sorts of muscles just to stay upright. Depending on your innate posture, this can aggravate a problem back. But wearing totally flat shoes can tip you the other way and be more tiring on the leg and low back muscles.

It is a good idea to change your shoes regularly. Varying the heel height (within reason) is good for your joints and muscles.

Q. Can I stop the exercises when my back feels better?

A. Most back problems develop slowly, so it follows that improving the state of your spine will also be slow – and ongoing. Your exercise regime has been carefully designed to appease your back when it is bad, and stretch and strengthen it when you are on the road to recovery. So don't be tempted to stop when your back starts feeling better. Your exercises will help you stay out of trouble and also keep you improving, so you are less likely to relapse.

Try to make the exercise session part of your daily routine. It should be something to look forward to; a few minutes of peace and quiet when you can draw in from the outside world and concentrate on yourself. Of course, when your back isn't bothering you as much, it won't hurt if you give the exercises a miss now and again (it is

unhealthy to become a slave to them!),
but regular sessions will continue to
improve the way your back works and its
overall health.

AND FINALLY ...

The Sarah Key Method is not a guarantee against back pain, but the information and exercises contained within these pages will help to fix most simple back problems.

Don't put up with back pain.

Persevere.
Be patient.
Take control of your back.

GOOD LUCK!

RESOURCES

The Sarah Key Method

To find an accredited practitioner of The Sarah Key Method (APSKM), go to: www.sarahkey.com

BackBlock

To purchase a wooden BackBlock, please send a cheque for £38 (price includes postage and packaging) to:
Blenheim Estate Office, Blenheim Palace, Woodstock, Oxfordshire, OX20 1PS, UK
(Please make cheques payable to Sunsar Blocks Limited. BackBlocks come with instructions that must be strictly followed.)

To purchase a BackBlock designed specially
for the Sarah Key System contact:
Back In Action
01494 434343
www.backinaction.co.uk/SarahKeyBackBlock

There are also Back In Action stores in
Central London, Bristol, Marlow and
Amersham, all of which stock BackBlocks, as
well as kneeling chairs, mattresses and back
supports. See www.backinaction.co.uk for
opening hours, maps and contact details.

INDEX